YOUR KNOWLEDGE HAS VALUE

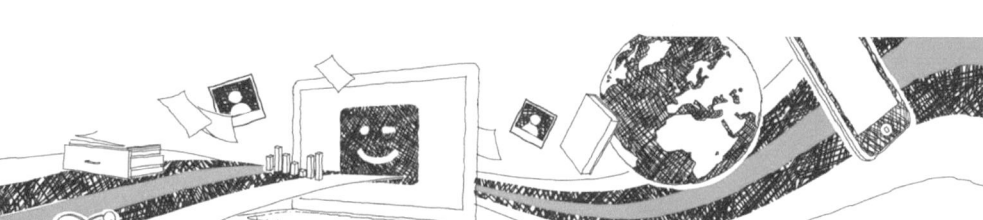

- We will publish your bachelor's and master's thesis, essays and papers

- Your own eBook and book - sold worldwide in all relevant shops

- Earn money with each sale

Upload your text at www.GRIN.com
and publish for free

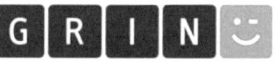

Bibliographic information published by the German National Library:

The German National Library lists this publication in the National Bibliography; detailed bibliographic data are available on the Internet at http://dnb.dnb.de .

This book is copyright material and must not be copied, reproduced, transferred, distributed, leased, licensed or publicly performed or used in any way except as specifically permitted in writing by the publishers, as allowed under the terms and conditions under which it was purchased or as strictly permitted by applicable copyright law. Any unauthorized distribution or use of this text may be a direct infringement of the author s and publisher s rights and those responsible may be liable in law accordingly.

Imprint:

Copyright © 2018 GRIN Verlag
Print and binding: Books on Demand GmbH, Norderstedt Germany
ISBN: 9783668627086

This book at GRIN:

https://www.grin.com/document/388323

Patrick Kimuyu

Mosquito Biology and Emerging Health Issues

GRIN Verlag

GRIN - Your knowledge has value

Since its foundation in 1998, GRIN has specialized in publishing academic texts by students, college teachers and other academics as e-book and printed book. The website www.grin.com is an ideal platform for presenting term papers, final papers, scientific essays, dissertations and specialist books.

Visit us on the internet:

http://www.grin.com/

http://www.facebook.com/grincom

http://www.twitter.com/grin_com

Mosquito Biology and Emerging Health Issues

Name: Patrick Kimuyu

Introduction

Mosquitoes remain to be among the most amazing organisms in the universe. Evolutionary data reveals that mosquitoes have survived for more than 30 million years in which 3,500 species have evolved. Despite the large genetic diversity observed in mosquitoes, only a few species have been found to bother humans. Over the years, research on mosquitoes has enabled entomologists in identifying different mosquito taxonomic classes. However, the classification of mosquitoes has been surrounded by unprecedented controversy because new species are being discovered year-by-year. The latest mosquito species to be identified include the two mosquito species belonging to the *Topomyia* genus recently discovered in Sri Lanka and the invasive *Aedes japonicas* species discovered in Asia (Kampen & Werner 2014).

According to the taxonomic classification, mosquitoes belong to the largest animal phylum; Arthropoda, and they are grouped in the Class: Insecta that comprises of other insects such as the flies. Down in the taxonomic classification, mosquitoes belong to the Order: Diptera and Family: Culicidae that comprise of various sub-families. At present, there are 43 known mosquito genera, which comprise of over 3,500 species (Rueda 2008).

In addition, an extensive study has been conducted to generate a comprehensive understanding on the anatomy, physiology and ecological characteristics of mosquitoes. It is believed that the ecological characteristics of mosquitoes and physiology are responsible for the emerging health issues. Therefore, this research paper will give a comprehensive overview of the mosquito biology. It will discuss the anatomy, physiology and ecological characteristics of mosquitoes. It will also provide a concise overview on the mosquito-borne diseases.

Mosquito Anatomy

Mosquitoes are two-winged insects with a small body which is divided into three principal body parts: the head, thorax and the abdomen (Byrd & Castner 2000). These body parts exhibit diverse anatomical features which define their biological functions. In general, an adult mosquito has a slender abdomen, and adults vary in length. Different mosquito species have different body lengths although their average length is estimated to be 6 mm, and 2.5 milligrams in weight.

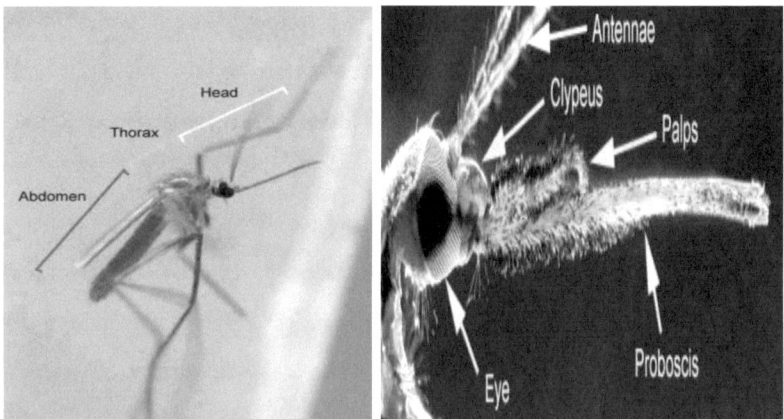

Figure: Mosquito body regions (University of Florida 2008 p.1-2)

Mosquitoes have a crammed head that contains sensory apparatus. These structures are believed to be the most significant anatomical features that define the feeding mode of mosquitoes. Some of the most significant anatomical apparatus found on the head region of mosquitoes are the eyes, antenna and the mouth parts. The two large compound eyes comprise of tiny lenses referred to as ommatidia which are concerned with the detection of movements. In addition to these sensory lenses in the compound eyes, mosquitoes possess simple photosensitive eyes known as the ocelli which are located on the top of their heads (Arikawa, Kawada, Takagi & Tatsuta 2006). These simple eyes are capable of detecting variations in light; thus, enabling mosquitoes in identifying their habitats.

The other sensory structures that are found on the head region are the antenna. The antennae are long feathery sensory organs that elongate forward from the head, and they contain sensitive receptors which enable mosquitoes to locate food sources. These receptors can detect chemicals such as carbon dioxide in human breath from as far as 100 feet. In addition, mosquitoes have other sensory structures such as the maxillary palp that is located between the antennae. This sensory apparatus is capable of detecting chemicals in the human sweat including urea and ocentol (Carde, Dekker & Geier 2005).

They also have a long serrated proboscis which holds the stylets used in piercing the skin and sucking blood. One of the tubes injects saliva into the animal's body from which the insect gets its blood meal, whereas the other stylet draws blood from the animal's blood vessels that lie underneath the skin (Kim, Kim & Lee 2010).

On the other hand, the thorax comprises of the appendages involved in the movement and locomotion of mosquitoes. The thorax in a torso connected to the head and it bears the three pairs of legs with tiny claws for grasping on surfaces and a pair of wings for flying. In addition to the wings, there are other small wing-like structures known as halteres which are used for steering during flight (Aldworth, Daniel, Fox & Hinterwirth 2012).

The slender abdomen hangs from the thorax, and it contains the digestive tract and respiratory structures. As such, it serves as the stomach; thus, it holds the blood meal. It also stores eggs in female mosquitoes. On the other hand, the abdomen contains small openings referred to as spiracles which are used for gaseous exchange.

In general, anatomical characteristics of mosquitoes are considered crucial in the taxonomic classification of mosquito species. For instance, the length of wings and the maxillary palp, as well as, the coloring and shape of the abdomen are used in identifying different species of mosquitoes.

Physiology in Mosquitoes

Physiological processes in mosquitoes exhibit differences among the species, although some of these differences are attributable to the adaptation of mosquitoes to various habitats and feeding modes.

Ordinarily, growth and development in mosquitoes involve three distinct stages which characterize their lifecycle. Mosquitoes' development is more or less the same as that observed in other holometabolous insects in which development involves the egg, larva, pupa and adult stages. Female mosquitoes lay eggs in aquatic environments through a process known as oviposition where they hatch into larval forms (Briegel 2003). The larva develops into a pupae form which in turn grows into adults in which males live for than a week whereas female mosquitoes have a lifespan of several weeks, especially in an environment with adequate supply of food sources.

Digestion in mosquitoes exhibits several characteristics that enable them to survive on their mode of feeding. Mosquitoes rely on plant juices and nectar as their principal sources of food, although female mosquitoes require a blood meal from birds and mammals for the development of eggs. It is worth noting that, male mosquitoes do not feed on blood as their female counterparts; instead, they feed on sugary plant juices for their nutrition. In female mosquitoes, blood is sucked from the animal skin through the use of a proboscis. During feeding, a mosquito injects anti-coagulant containing saliva into the host's tissue fluid and draws it into the gut where digestive enzymes including proteases breakdown the blood meal for absorption. Thereafter, waste products that include uric acid are excreted through the anus.

Gaseous exchange in mosquitoes occurs through the tracheal system which comprises of the spiracles located on both sides of the abdomen. The tracheal system contains end bulbs or air sacs which are in contact with the coelomic fluids in the surrounding body tissues. Therefore, respiratory gases, oxygen and carbon dioxide enter and leave the tracheal system through diffusion in which oxygen is taken up for respiration and carbon dioxide exhaled as a by-product.

Moreover, mosquitoes have an elaborate endocrine system that controls the release of hormones. These hormones are believed to play a significant role in defining the behavior of mosquitoes.

Ecological Role of Mosquitoes

Distribution of Mosquitoes

From an ecological perspective, mosquitoes exhibit a widespread distribution in which they colonize all ecological zones except the Antarctica region. Ordinarily, mosquitoes are abundant in the tropical regions which are characterized by warm and humid climatic conditions. These climatic conditions are favorable for the reproduction of mosquitoes, and this explains why most mosquito species are found within the tropical regions where they remain active throughout the year. In temperate regions, mosquitoes are believed to hibernate over winter and re-emerge during summer. In general, mosquitoes live in aquatic and damp habitats in which larvae and pupae forms live predominantly in aquatic habitats, whereas adults are free flying and they prefer cool or damp places (Alto & Jusot 2011).

Ecological Role of Mosquitoes in the Ecosystem

Mosquitoes are believed to play a significant role in the ecosystem. One of the most principal ecological roles played by mosquitoes is the connection of food chains that help in maintaining energy cycles in the ecosystem. Some of the beneficial impacts of mosquitoes include providing food to predatory aquatic animals such as fish which feeds on mosquito larvae. On the other hand, adult mosquitoes serve as principal sources of food for bats, birds and other arthropods such as spiders and dragonflies.

However, it is worth noting that mosquitoes have both positive and negative impacts on the ecosystem. They serve as disease vectors in which they transmit pathogens through bites. Some of the pathogens transmitted by mosquitoes cause devastating health consequences leading to animal deaths and economic losses (Juliano & Lounibos 2005).

Emerging Health issues

Mosquitoes are believed to be vectors for various parasites which cause diseases in humans and other animals. Some of the common mosquito-borne diseases include malaria, dengue fever, yellow fever and encephalitis.

Malaria

Malaria is one of the life-threatening infectious diseases whose impacts are experienced in the U.S. healthcare system. Its prevalence reached the highest level in 2011 since 1971. However, most U.S. residents acquired the disease from tropical countries where it is endemic. Epidemiological reports indicate that 70% of malaria cases in 2011were acquired from tropical countries, primarily in Africa (O'Meara, Mangeni, Steketee & Greenwood 2010).

Ordinarily, malaria is caused by Plasmodium parasite and its transmission occurs through the bites of infected *Anopheles* mosquitoes (Autino, Castel, Noris & Russo 2012). The parasite undergoes two successive asexual replication stages in the human body and infects red blood cells where it produces toxins (Critchlow, Staves & Watt 2007). The first stage involves the parasite's multiplication in the liver and then it enters the blood circulation where it infects the erythrocytes causing hemolytic reactions.

Characteristics of malaria include headache, fever and vomiting. However, it is worth noting that these characteristics occur within 10 to 15 days after the bite of an infected *Anopheles* mosquito. In addition, malaria symptoms occur depending on multiplication stages involved in the liver and blood circulation (WHO, 2013). For instance, chills are manifested during the exoerythrocytic cycle in which the parasite becomes infectious. It is believed that the destruction of the erythrocytes interferes with the blood supply to various body organs leading to the general body weakness (Westenberger et al. 2010). In most cases, untreated malaria becomes life-threatening after the disruption of the blood circulation in the body in which vital organs lack adequate blood supply.

Malaria was eliminated in the U.S. in 1951 through the adoption of the appropriate epidemiological models designed by CDC. However, malaria cases increased significantly by 1971 (Cotter et al. 2013).

In the US, prevalence rates remained low until 2011 when malaria cases increased to as high as 1,925. This was estimated to be a 14% increase from the previous year, and it was the highest incidence rate since 1941. Currently, the burden of malaria on the U.S. healthcare systems is relatively high owing to the 2011 disease outcomes. Despite the low mortality rate reported in the U.S., the country has been spending large sums of money in funding government health initiatives. Moreover, malaria surveillance in the U.S. consumes a large percentage of healthcare expenditure, primarily in monitoring imported malaria cases from endemic regions and responding to outbreaks as it was the case in 2011 (Doudou et al. 2012).

Globally, the prevalence trends of malaria seem to have changed significantly leading to an increase in malaria related morbidities. Recent epidemiological studies indicate that the global deaths from malaria increased to 3.3 billion in 2010 from 0.8 billion deaths recorded in 1900 (Autino, Castel, Noris & Russo 2012). Therefore, it is apparent that, malaria poses a significant threat to mankind, and this threat is intensified by the emerging health issues surrounding malaria transmission such as the discovery of new malaria transmitting mosquito species and insecticide resistance by Anopheles mosquitoes (Breman, McKenzie & O'Meara 2005).

Dengue Fever

Another mosquito-borne disease which has raised health concerns is the dengue fever, a serious arboviral disease which occurs in Asia, America and Africa. This disease is transmitted by *Aedes albopictus* and *Ae. aegypti*. It is reported that, the incidence rate of dengue fever has been rising since 2000 in which 600 deaths have been recorded in Indonesia.

On the other hand, yellow fever is increasingly becoming a threat in tropical regions in which an estimation of 30,000 deaths is reported in 33 countries, yearly. In 2003, 226 cases of yellow fever were reported in America, whereas 27 deaths occurred in South Sudan in which 178 cases were reported.

West Nile Virus

Moreover, new cases of the West Nile Virus infections in different parts of the world have increased the harm caused by mosquitoes on other animals. This disease virus undergoes its lifecycle in birds and mosquitoes in which it is transmitted to humans and other mammals such as horses through mosquito bites. Since its discovery in 1937, the West Nile Virus has been causing deaths in birds and wild mammals, but its infection has spread to humans. In 1999, the West Nile virus was reported to cause 7 human deaths in North America, and its prevalence among humans has increased significantly whereby it has spread to most states in the US. Evidence shows that, the West Nile virus had caused 1.5 million infections in the US by 2010.

Conclusion

In a brief conclusion, it is apparent that mosquitoes exhibit diverse features of interest to entomologists, as well as, epidemiologists. The biology of mosquitoes is relatively different from that of other insects because; some mosquito species have been implicated in some of the emerging health issues. For instance, mosquitoes have been identified to be significant disease vectors. In theory, the vector role of mosquitoes is attributable to their anatomical and physiological features which enable them to adapt in virtually all ecological zones. One of the most significant ecological benefits of mosquitoes is the maintenance of energy cycles in the ecosystem where they serve as food sources for predatory animals such as fish and bats. However, mosquitoes cause devastating health and economic impacts on humans because they act as vectors for pathogens which cause diseases in humans and other animals.

References

Aldworth, Z, Daniel, T, Fox, J & Hinterwirth, A 2012, *Chapter 19: Insect inertial measurement units - gyroscopic sensing of body rotation*, New York, NY: Springer.

Alto, O & Jusot, J 2011, Short term effect of rainfall on suspected malaria episodes at Magaria, Niger: a time series study, *Trans R Soc Trop Med Hyg*. vol. 105, pp. 637-643.

Arikawa, K, Kawada, H, Takagi, M & Tatsuta, H 2006, Comparative study on the relationship between photoperiodic host-seeking behavioral patterns and the eye parameters of mosquitoes, *Journal of Insect Physiology*, vol. 52. no. 1, pp. 67–75.

Autino, B, Castel, F, Noris, A & Russo, R 2012, Epidemiology of Malaria in Endemic Areas, *Mediterr J Hematol Infect Dis*, vol. 4. no. 1, pp. 1-10, viewed 16 Jan 2018, <http://www.mjhid.org/article/view/10960/html>

Breman, G, McKenzie, F & O'Meara, W 2005, The promise and potential challenges of intermittent preventive treatment for malaria in infants (IPTi), *Malaria Journal*, vol. 4, pp. 33.

Briegel, H 2003, Physiological bases of mosquito ecology, *J Vector Ecol*. vol. 28, no. 1, pp. 1-11.

Byrd, J & Castner, L 2000, *Forensic entomology: the utility of arthropods in legal investigations*, Boca Raton, Fl: CRC Press.

Carde, R, Dekker, T & Geier, M 2005, Carbon dioxide instantly sensitizes female yellow fever mosquitoes to human skin odors, *The Journal of Experimental Biology*, vol. 208, pp. 2963-2972.

Cotter, C. et al 2013, The changing epidemiology of malaria elimination: new strategies for new challenges, *Lancet*, vol. 382, pp. 900.

Critchlow, A, Staves, J & Watt, C 2007, *Malaria vaccines*, viewed 13 Jan 2018, <http://www.stanford.edu/class/humbio153/MalariaVac/index.html>

Doudou, H et al 2012, A refined estimate of the malaria burden in Niger, *Malaria Journal*, vol. 11, pp. 89.

Juliano, S & Lounibos, L 2005, Ecology of invasive mosquitoes: effects on resident species and on human health, *Ecology Letters*, vol. 8. no. 5, pp. 558–560.

Kampen, H & Werner, D 2014, Out of the bush: the Asian bush mosquito Aedes japonicus japonicus (Theobald, 1901) (Diptera, Culicidae) becomes invasive, *Parasit Vectors*, vol. 7, pp. 59. Viewed 16 Jan 2018, <http://www.ncbi.nlm.nih.gov/pmc/articles/PMC3917540/>

Kim, H, Kim, B & Lee, S 2010, Experimental analysis of the blood-sucking mechanism of female mosquitoes, *The Journal of Experimental Biology,* vol. 214, pp. 1163-1169.

O'Meara, P, Mangeni, N, Steketee, R & Greenwood, B 2010, Changes in the burden of malaria in sub-Saharan Africa, *Lancet Infect Dis.*, vol. 10, pp. 545-555.

Rueda, L 2008, Golbal diversity of mosquitoes (Insecta: Diptera: Culicidae) in freshwater, *Hydrobiologia*, vol. 595, pp. 477-487.

University of Florida 2008, Basic Adult Anatomy, viewed 12 Jan 2018, <http://fmel.ifas.ufl.edu/key/anatomy/adult.shtml>

Westenberger, S et al. (2010) A systems-based analysis of plasmodium vivax lifecycle transcription from human to mosquito*, PLoS Negl Trop Dis* vol. 4. no. 4, pp. e653.

WHO 2013, *Malaria*, viewed 16 Jan 2018, <http://www.who.int/topics/malaria/en/ >

YOUR KNOWLEDGE HAS VALUE

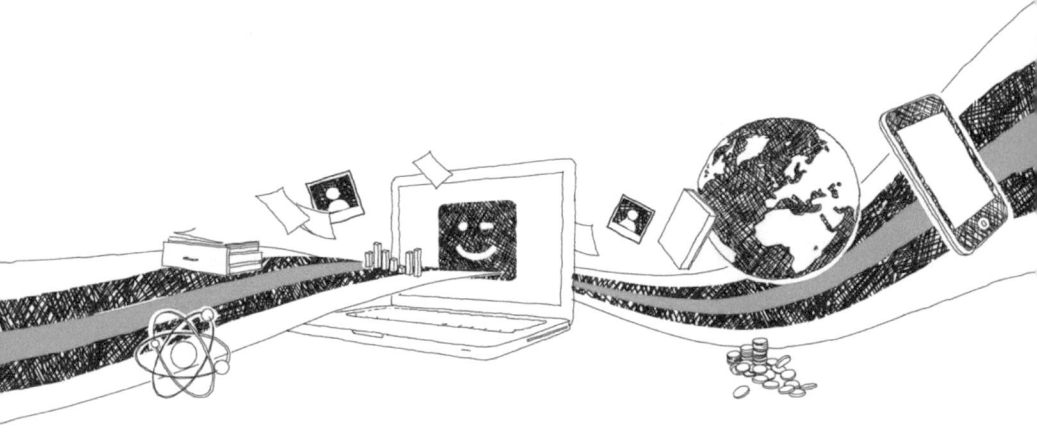

- We will publish your bachelor's and master's thesis, essays and papers

- Your own eBook and book - sold worldwide in all relevant shops

- Earn money with each sale

Upload your text at www.GRIN.com
and publish for free

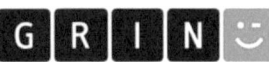